POCKET GUIDES
FOR NURSING AND HEALTH CARE

CW00820323

BREAKING
BAD NEWS

A unique series of pocket-sized books designed to help healthcare students

"All the information was clear and concise, this book is exactly what I was looking for." ★★★★★

"A great little guide. All the basic information needed to have a quick reference." ★★★★★

"A very useful, well-written and practical pocket book." ★★★★★

"Written by students for students. A must for any student about to head on placement." ★★★★★

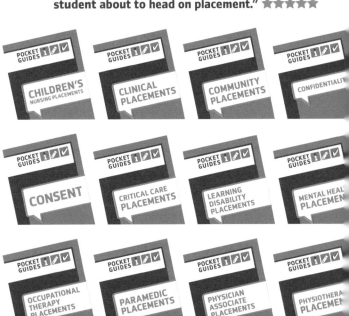

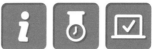
BREAKING BAD NEWS

Gillian Oakley

University of Central Lancashire

Lantern

ISBN 9781914962189
First published in 2024 by Lantern Publishing Ltd

Lantern Publishing Limited, The Old Hayloft, Vantage
Business Park, Bloxham Road, Banbury OX16 9UX, UK
www.lanternpublishing.com

British Library Cataloguing in Publication Data
A catalogue record for this book is available from the British Library

The authors and publisher have made every attempt to ensure
the content of this book is up to date and accurate. However,
healthcare knowledge and information is changing all the time
so the reader is advised to double-check any information in
this text on drug usage, treatment procedures, the use of
equipment, etc. to confirm that it complies with the latest safety
recommendations, standards of practice and legislation, as well as
local Trust policies and procedures. Students are advised to check
with their tutor and/or practice supervisor before carrying out
any of the procedures in this textbook.

Typeset by Medlar Publishing Solutions Pvt Ltd, India
Printed and bound in the UK

Last digit is the print number: 10 9 8 7 6 5 4 3 2 1

Personal information

Name: . . . .

Contact number: . . . .

University contact details: . . . .

. . . .

. . . .

. . . .

Personal tutor details: . . . .

CONTACT IN CASE OF EMERGENCY

Name: . . . .

Contact number: . . . .

Contents

Preface

This book builds on and updates the work by Peter Kaye (1996), who developed a ten-step approach to breaking bad news. Kaye's original pocketbook was published in 1996 and at the time he acknowledged that communication skills training was limited. Since then, there have been a variety of communication skills training programmes developed and rolled out across care settings including SAGE & THYME (Connolly *et al.*, 2010) and Advanced Communication Skills workshops (Fallowfield *et al.*, 2002), to name but two.

This easy-to-use pocket guide has been designed for any healthcare practitioner or clinician to use in any healthcare setting.

A new model/mnemonic as an aide-memoire is introduced to assist clinicians when delivering bad news to patients, relatives, or significant others. SUPPORTS stands for

S: Set the scene

U: Understand the patient's perspective

P: Prepare the patient (fire a warning shot)

P: Pass on the information

O: Observe silence

R: Respect and respond to emotion

T: Time for questions and clarification

S: Summary and close

Gillian Oakley

About the author

Gillian Oakley qualified as a nurse in 1995 and is a university lecturer at the University of Central Lancashire (UCLan) and an Advanced Clinical Practitioner (ACP) in Palliative Care. She teaches postgraduate courses in palliative care, cancer care, acute oncology, non-medical prescribing, advanced clinical practice and end-of-life care. Gillian is also an advanced communication skills trainer for the connected programme.

Prior to joining UCLan in 2016, Gillian worked for 14 years as a Macmillan CNS before completing the ACP training in 2014. She is currently undertaking a Professional Doctorate in health sciences, on communication and consultation models utilised in practice.

Gillian is a clinical trustee of Pendleside Hospice in Lancashire and maintains a strong link to clinical practice. Her interest in breaking bad news is motivated by stories from patients who have given accounts of being given bad news poorly and the subsequent negative impact of this.

Introduction

Breaking bad news is a common cause of anxiety for doctors, nurses and allied health professionals (Francis and Robertson, 2023) and yet having to give news and information to patients that could be seen as bad news is a common occurrence in health care. This pocket guide is written for any healthcare professional who is required to break bad news to patients, their loved ones and or even colleagues.

When we think about bad news, we sometimes wrongly assume that this is telling a patient that they have some life-changing or untreatable condition; however, bad news can come in many forms. The principles outlined within this book can be applied to many situations when bad news needs to be delivered.

This guide outlines a new model and mnemonic, SUPPORTS, that will assist practitioners and provide an easy-to-follow framework. Although this book introduces a new model for clinicians to follow, it must be stressed that each communication situation is different and requires clinicians to have a flexible approach and respond to the patient's emotions and concerns throughout the process.

Each chapter addresses a separate concept, including a discussion around what constitutes bad news, why it is important to deliver bad news well, why it is difficult to deliver bad news, and how not to deliver bad news. Finally we will look at how to apply the new model using the new mnemonic SUPPORTS. Also included are examples from practice to support each concept, as well as references to supporting literature.

1 | What is bad news?

Bad news has been defined as anything that will potentially change an individual's plans or affect outcomes or 'vision for the future' (Kaye, 2023). For example, someone being told that they have a cancer diagnosis is the obvious situation that healthcare professionals would consider as bad news; however, for some people finding out that their train has been cancelled, that an appointment has been delayed or test results have been lost (plus many others), is bad news. Fallowfield and Jenkins (2004) support this, stating that bad news can be seen as any bad, sad or significant information which impacts negatively on a person's views or expectations of their present and future. Healthcare practitioners need to respect that something they may consider as being insignificant to an individual, might be perceived by the recipient as being significant, and can be devastating. Buckman (1984) identifies that bad news for patients can be any information that produces negative expectations about their future.

 Examples of what bad news could be:

- *"You cannot visit outside the hours of 5pm to 8pm."*
- *"Your appointment has been cancelled."*
- *"You have cancer."*
- *"We have lost your scan results."*
- *"The treatment will have side-effects."*
- *"There is a waiting period of 4 weeks for that investigation."*
- *"You have developed diabetes."*
- *"There are no appointments available until next week."*

This is not an exhaustive list.

As you can see from the examples listed above, bad news can be any number of things and is individual to the receiver.

As deliverers of bad news, we need to consider ways in which we can plan and prepare ourselves to give information in a manner that reduces the risk of misinterpretation or misunderstanding, as well as being able to demonstrate empathy and compassion and deal with the emotion of the recipient. Added to this is the sense of professionalism we achieve by knowing we have done a difficult job well.

One of the challenges we face quite often as healthcare providers is that we may only have known the patient for a few minutes or hours; therefore, a trusting relationship may not yet have been established (Monden et al., 2016). In order to facilitate the building of an effective therapeutic relationship in a short period of time, the new model outlined in this book offers a structured format to aid our communication skills when delivering bad news. That being said, for situations when we have already established a relationship with a patient, the new model offers an approach that encourages healthcare professionals to continue to build upon that, by enabling the practitioner to give bad news in an empathetic manner.

Breaking bad news is everyone's business. Changes within the NHS and health care have resulted in more levels of responsibility for staff members who in previous decades would not have been expected to deliver bad news. In previous times, the giving of bad news was reserved for senior medics. However, with the development of advanced roles such as Advanced Clinical Practitioner and Clinical Nurse Specialist, the task of breaking bad news also falls to many other staff groups.

'Bad news' comes in many forms, as discussed previously. Therefore all staff should have the ability to deliver bad news and give information in a professional and empathetic manner. There may be practitioners who feel that the giving of bad news is not part of their current role. It could be argued that all staff, irrespective of grade, will deliver some form of information that patients and/or relatives may perceive as bad news. Equally, as a healthcare practitioner's career progresses, the level of information and responsibility to deliver bad news may become a requirement, therefore it is worth having the knowledge and understanding of how to do it well, in order to be prepared in advance.

Scenario from clinical practice

A newly qualified Operating Department Practitioner (ODP) is recovering a patient who was taken to theatre for an emergency operation due to bowel perforation. The surgeon was required to form a temporary colostomy in order to save the bowel. The patient was told prior to surgery that there was a possibility that they may need a temporary colostomy fitting but that the surgeon was going to try to avoid this if possible. Upon waking, the patient asked the ODP what surgery was done. The ODP was required to deliver the information to the patient that a colostomy had been formed. For the patient this may be classed as bad news.

You can see from the above example that the ODP had a duty of care to tell the patient, as the surgeon was not available. The requirement was for the ODP to inform the patient in a sensitive and compassionate manner.

Why is it important to break bad news well?

When bad news is given poorly it can cause distress to patients and their loved ones, and is one of the largest factors cited in complaints to the NHS (NHS Digital, 2022). Delivering bad news can also affect the news-giver, with Edwards (2010) suggesting that if it goes badly, this can cause distress and anxiety to the healthcare professional and can impact upon job satisfaction and confidence.

As mentioned in *Chapter 1*, within health care it is important that we build and maintain therapeutic relationships with our patients. Before we consider the reasons for this, we first need to identify what a therapeutic relationship is.

2.1 The importance of a therapeutic relationship

The importance of building a trusting relationship between patients and clinicians has been well publicised and advocated throughout multiple core texts within health care, and is seen as the 'backbone of nursing practice' (Moreno-Poyato and Rodríguez-Nogueira, 2021).

But what is a 'therapeutic relationship'? The concept is difficult to define. However, the principles of trust, patient satisfaction, honesty, empathy and respect are linked to the concept (Greenhalgh and Heath, 2010). Epstein *et al.* (2000) define the therapeutic relationship as the nurses' ability to consciously use their personality to get close to the patient to be able to perform any nursing interventions effectively. They go on to suggest that clinicians are required to be self-conscious, self-aware, and to have a philosophy about life, death and the overall human situation.

So how does a clinician build or demonstrate a therapeutic relationship?

Mirhaghi *et al.* (2017) suggest that the therapeutic relationship is composed of 'significant knowing' and 'meaningful connectedness', arguing that knowing your patient is the main element and that a relationship can only be built if a clinician has knowledge of the patient and what the effect of disease is on that person. It could be suggested that being curious is a starting point. Be curious as to how the patient is feeling, thinking or experiencing a situation. Spiers and Wood (2010) suggest this is 'being in the moment' with another human, utilising interpersonal skills such as listening to the narrative of the patient and interpreting meaning.

Think about the reasons why you chose health care as your career. Aside from financial remuneration, it is arguable that most clinicians choose to work in health care to care for people. How do you do this? What do you do each day that demonstrates to your patients that you care?

Working in health care can be stressful, frustrating, rewarding and many other things, but every now and again, take your thoughts back to why you came into health care in the first place. This exercise will enable you to consider how and why we strive to build therapeutic relationships with our patients.

Make your own notes here.

_____

_____

_____

_____

Within health care it is important that we build and maintain therapeutic relationships with our patients for the following reasons:

1. **Duty of care.** Gone are the days when doctors held back information because 'it was in the patient's best interest'. UK policy and law, such as the Human Rights Act (1998), the Mental Capacity Act (2005) and the Health and Social Care Act (2014), plus adhering to ethical principles of autonomy, non-maleficence, beneficence and justice, ensures that patients and their loved ones are informed regarding diagnoses and treatment options. The challenge is ensuring this news is delivered in a compassionate manner.

2. **To build and maintain trust.** The building of therapeutic relationships is paramount to effective care. We want patients to feel they can discuss their concerns and divulge information that sometimes can be sensitive. It is difficult to help patients if we do not have all the information from them in the first instance. An example may be that a patient reports one concern, but they then report another right at the end of an appointment. It may be that the later issue was the real reason for speaking with you, but they required confidence to raise this. Patient-centred care underpins the philosophy of good health care (NICE, 2021).

3. **To promote concordance.** Evidence and research confirm that if we have a therapeutic relationship with our patients, they are more likely to follow treatment plans that have been developed using shared decision-making. This can only be achieved if patients have all the information, even if it is bad news. A concordant relationship is based upon trust and although strongly linked to compliance within the literature, it is characterised by patient-centredness rather than a

paternalistic approach. It is also linked to autonomy and patient participation in shared decision-making.

4. **To empower and inform.** Reducing uncertainty and having knowledge about their situation enables patients to adjust to the reality. The withholding of bad news or information can lead to many adverse consequences such as the patient making poor clinical decisions. An example would be a patient choosing to undergo a life-altering surgery without being given all the information regarding consequences. Honesty matters to patients (Calnan and Rowe, 2008).

5. **To allow for realistic planning.** Having 'all' of the information, even if it is upsetting, enables patients to make informed choices about their future, facilitates realistic planning and allows honest communication with family and loved ones.

Notes

Advance care planning

Advance care planning is a concept that encourages patients to communicate with healthcare professionals and their loved ones regarding their wishes at end of life, such as what they do and do not want. Although upsetting to be told they have a limited amount of time to live, having this information allows for planning and putting affairs in order such as writing a will, and minimises the risk of missed opportunities to say or do things that are important to that individual.

Some patients may be able to access life insurance or other financial benefits such as early retirement or mortgage support if they have received a life-limiting diagnosis. Having the information allows a patient to start the process of 'putting their affairs in order' or accessing financial support.

Patients who are told that they are required to have prolonged treatment over a long period of time, and what the implications of this are, will be able to communicate with employers, family etc. to ensure they access appropriate support.

A final thought to end this chapter: the principles of the 6 Cs (NHS England, 2012) can be applied to the practice of breaking bad news.

The 6 Cs of care

- Care
- Compassion
- Competence
- Communication
- Courage
- Commitment

3

Why is it difficult to break bad news well?

The giving of bad news has been identified as a cause of high stress levels, with healthcare practitioners reporting that it is something they feel underprepared to do well (Almaguer et al., 2017). It may also lead to burnout (Cheon et al., 2017).

There are multiple factors that make communication and breaking bad news difficult.

Here they are broken into four categories of barriers and challenges (Norouzinia et al., 2015; Heaven and Maguire, 1997; Cheon et al., 2017). The table below depicts common (although by no means exhaustive) themes, aspects of which are then discussed in more detail section by section.

Barriers and challenges associated with delivering bad news

Factors between healthcare professionals and patients	Colloquial language differences
	Cultural differences
	Gender differences
	Inability to connect with the patient
	Individual relationships with the patient (known for a long time)
Environmental factors	Lack of space and privacy
	Lack of time
	Interruptions
	Relevant people absent
	Conflict within a team

Professional-related factors	Fear of upsetting the patient
	Own beliefs
	Unable to address/answer questions
	Being uncertain
	Feeling unsupported
	Lack of understanding of the patient's needs
	Lack of training
	Being overworked
Patient-related factors	Struggling with words
	Literacy levels
	Poor understanding
	Lack of information
	Mental capacity issues
	Physical challenges
	Feeling unsupported
	Relevant people absent
	Physical symptoms, such as pain

3.1 Factors between healthcare professionals and patients

As healthcare professionals we are encouraged to form a trusting, therapeutic relationship with our patients, where patients can express concerns and ask questions. However, there are several factors that potentially hinder this. From a patient's perspective, Neelima *et al.* (2020) suggest that past unpleasant experiences and the use of medical jargon can cause barriers to the building of a therapeutic relationship with a clinician.

Scenario from clinical practice

A patient was told that they had had an 'MI'.

Their response was, "Thank God that's all it was, I thought I was having a heart attack."

Within health care we use many acronyms and abbreviations throughout our working day; however, patients quite often don't know what they mean and can feel uncomfortable asking.

Careful consideration needs to be given to the words we use, as often these can be misinterpreted. An example is when we talk about death and dying. For a variety of reasons, we sometimes may feel uncomfortable using the words 'death' and 'dying' so we try to soften the blow by using colloquial language (euphemisms) such as 'passed' or 'gone to sleep'. The problem with some of these phrases is that they may be misinterpreted.

Scenario from clinical practice

An 8-year-old child was told that his father had 'gone to sleep', rather than being told he had died. A few months later the child needed to go for surgery and required a general anaesthetic. The nurse explained to the child that the doctor would put some "special medicine" into his arm so he would just "go to sleep". The child was extremely distressed because he thought he was not going to wake up. It is easy to see that the clinician had good intentions when using the term 'gone to sleep' but it can be seen why this was misinterpreted later.

A patient attended an oncology appointment and asked *"How long have I got?"*. The doctor replied *"only four weeks"*. The patient was extremely distressed and upset. Upon exploration, the patient had wanted to know how long she had left to live, but the doctor thought she was asking how long she had left on chemotherapy.

You can see from the above examples how poor communication impacted upon the experiences of these two individuals.

We live in a multicultural society and talk to colleagues and patients from different cultural backgrounds daily. For some patients, English may not be their first language and as a result they may have strong accents which might lead to miscommunication; this can sometimes be the case with regional accents too. It can sometimes feel embarrassing asking someone to repeat what they have said due to us not understanding; however, it is important to clarify and understand fully.

A healthcare professional may have attempted to deliver bad news in the past and this experience went badly, resulting in a lack of confidence and reticence or reluctance when attempting this again.

Another factor which may impact on the communication between patients and healthcare professionals is that a patient's situation may be like that of a health professional's personal experience, making it difficult to connect. For example, a healthcare professional who has experienced the death of a parent or loved one due to a particular illness may find it challenging to engage with a terminally ill patient with a similar diagnosis, due to fear that it will stir difficult memories and emotions.

"I avoided the patient in bed 3 because she reminded me of my own mum and when she was dying. I just couldn't face telling her that her surgery had been cancelled because I knew that I would struggle to keep my emotions in check" (a fictitious example of when personal experiences interfere with a clinician's professional role).

Having an awareness of one's own bias and attitudes helps healthcare professionals to start addressing these when we plan to have difficult conversations with our patients.

> **Scenario from clinical practice**
>
> A patient decided against having curative chemotherapy, knowing that without it, they would die from the cancer. The nurse looking after the patient has been told her mum couldn't have any more chemotherapy because she wasn't well enough. The nurse struggled to talk with the patient as she was angry that someone would refuse treatment when her mum had been told she couldn't have any more.

3.2 Environmental factors

Many of the clinical areas where we deliver patient care are busy, noisy and not very private. When we are giving bad news, this can cause barriers to effective communication. As we will see later in the book, clinicians are encouraged to be prepared. This includes taking into consideration where we give bad news.

For example, it is not best practice or appropriate to give sensitive information knowing that there is only a curtain between patients. This can be a barrier to patients who may have questions but don't want to ask, knowing other patients or visitors can hear them. Equally, if a patient is emotionally distressed, there is little dignity when privacy is not considered.

Another factor cited by healthcare professionals is patient–staff ratios, linking with the concept that staff feel unable to afford patients time, and therefore avoid engaging in conversations due to fear that they will not have time to deal with any problems. However, research has shown that it is possible for effective communication to be done, and done well, in a short period of time (Wilkinson *et al*, 2008).

 Other barriers

- Interruptions from phones, pagers and other electronic devices
- Lack of space away from other people who are present, but who might inhibit the conversation, e.g. relatives, colleagues, students
- People not being available who need to be there to allow a discussion to take place, e.g. relatives, colleagues.

3.3 Professional factors

Many healthcare professionals report that they have not had much formal communication skills training, or that they lack the confidence to communicate well. As a result, they avoid communicating with patients, or they do it badly, through fear of not being able to support the patient well or deal with the potential upset or anger.

Such fears can include the following:

- Fear of unleashing strong emotions, e.g. anger, uncontrollable tears, expressions of horror, screaming.

- Fear of upsetting the patient or relative; saying something which might upset the person or make them lose control.
- Fear of damaging the person and causing more harm than good by saying the wrong thing, by forcing someone to face something or by giving too much information.
- Fear of adding to the person's difficulties and making the situation worse for the person.
- Fear of saying the wrong thing to the person because you are unsure that you have fully understood yourself, if the information is complex and difficult to explain, or if you yourself have strong beliefs about certain approaches to the situation.
- Fear of a person's refusal to accept your opinion, and potentially refuse life-saving treatments.
- Fear of taking up too much time by opening up the 'can of worms' in a busy clinic by triggering someone to break down and cry, or by entering into a complex conversation when time is limited.
- Feeling that there is no support or referral pathway for the person when problems are identified, i.e. having nowhere you can refer the person to for additional help.
- Conflict with the team, meaning that emotional energy you might invest in the patient is spent watching your own back or helping others in the team.

Although this list of fears and concerns is not exhaustive, as each healthcare professional will have their own thoughts and feelings, the new mnemonic highlighted in *Chapter 5* aims to assist clinicians to deliver bad news well and as a result alleviate these fears.

3.4 Patient-related factors

Patient barriers to effective communication can be obvious factors such as physical disabilities, language barriers, not understanding the terminology that healthcare practitioners use, or poor literacy and/or mental capacity. The patient is more than likely to be anxious in the context of receiving bad news and anxiety stimulates the stress response, which shuts down the capacity to process information.

We know from research that anxious patients often only hear the first and last thing they are told (Murdock, 1962; Glanzer and Cunitz, 1966). All the other bits of information are lost, resulting in poor understanding.

Some patients aren't ready to hear bad news. Patients are often said to be 'in denial'. This 'denial' is a valid coping mechanism that healthcare professionals need to acknowledge and explore further with the patient. The way to do this is addressed in *Section 5.11*.

Some fears that patients may have include:

- Fear of being stigmatised for admitting to the illness or the ability to cope with it. There is still a culture amongst some people that illness always results from poor lifestyle choices. This often leads to stigmas being associated with certain types of illness, e.g. lung cancer, cervical cancer, HIV/AIDS, etc.
- Fear of losing control and breaking down. Patients and also their relatives worry about losing control, breaking down or crying in front of professionals. Many people are very private and might never have cried in front of anybody outside of their closest family and friendship circle.
- Fear of having their worst fears confirmed.
- Fear of burdening the healthcare professional. Patients are often heard saying that they didn't want to bother the doctor or the nurse because they can see they are busy. Perceiving we have limited time acts as a barrier to effective communication. There is an increasing amount of evidence to show that patients and relatives worry about

the burden to the health professionals who care for them. They are very aware of how busy health professionals are and express concerns about taking up too much time or overwhelming the professionals with the breadth of their worries or questions.

- Fear of burdening family or loved ones. Patients often worry about the impact of their illness on their families. There is significant evidence to show that they protect their loved ones from knowing about their concerns and worries, and that they worry about being a burden to them (Fox, 2021).

In the next chapter we will look at how not to break bad news, before coming on to a new model to help you break bad news well in *Chapter 5*.

✏️ **Notes**

4   How not to break bad news

In this chapter we will consider the impact of breaking bad news poorly, and explore how not to give bad news.

In the following case scenarios we will see there are many barriers and challenges associated with giving bad news, and as a result we hear of many examples from patients of when bad news was given poorly. This chapter explores some of the ways in which bad news has been given poorly and incorporates some examples from practice. The scenarios are based on real-life experiences that have been reported by patients, but the presentation has been generalised and fictionalised to protect patient anonymity.

4.1 Impact on patients when done badly

Many healthcare professionals, when asked, will say they have witnessed bad news being delivered poorly. When we consider what the impact of this is on the patient, there is no doubt that this varies from patient to patient based upon their individual personalities and resilience. However, from my own clinical experience, patients talk about the distress caused by being given bad news poorly or delivered in an unempathetic way.

 Time to think

> Think of a time when you have experienced a patient being given bad news poorly. Write your own notes here on what the impact was for the patient and what factors influenced the way the news was given.
>
> _____
>
> _____
>
> _____

Case scenarios

Patient: *"The doctor just blurted it out that I had weeks to live and that they were referring me to the hospice. I wasn't prepared to hear it. I had no idea things were so bad. I was on my own in a hospital bed and she just walked away. I remember feeling overwhelmed and frightened. I just sat there and cried on my own."*

In this example you can see there was no thought or planning when delivering this news to the patient. Following on from this experience the patient then had to pass on the news to her family without any support from healthcare professionals. There was no opportunity for asking questions or clarification. Not only was the patient distressed, but the wider impact on her family was marked.

Patient: *"I answered the phone at 10pm and a person on the other end said, 'I'm sorry but your father has just died, can you come in?'. They didn't even introduce themselves. I knew my father was poorly, but I wasn't expecting him to die."*

In this example the caller made no attempt to build a therapeutic relationship with the family member or prepare them. They should have introduced themselves in the first instance and fired a warning shot that they were calling with bad news. Factors that influenced the caller may be that they assumed the family member was aware, or that they didn't have the skill set to perform this activity well.

Patient: *"The doctor told me I was going to lose my leg, but he didn't even look up from his notes when he told me. I felt utterly devastated... how was I going to cope? I'm a single parent with three young children. I was left lying there in disbelief wondering if it was all just a nightmare. The doctor was abrupt and just walked away."*

In these general examples, there was little planning in the delivery of the bad news. There was limited patient-centredness and empathy. We cannot assume that we know or understand the impact of bad news on patients, but effective communication can aid the building of a therapeutic relationship.

The following examples highlight specific ways in which bad news can be delivered badly. As you read through them, think about the impact on the patient of receiving bad news in these ways.

4.2 Inappropriate communication channel

> **Clinician (telephone call):** *"Hello, is that Mrs Smith? I'm one of the doctors at the health centre. Your results have come back, and I can confirm you have cancer."*

In this example there was no planning or consideration given to the delivery of the bad news. The giving of bad news ideally should be done face to face. There may be circumstances when other communication channels such as telephones are necessary; however, this should not be the norm and should be avoided if possible when delivering bad news. As a starting point the doctor did not introduce themselves by name and there was no attempt by the doctor to establish what the patient knew already.

4.3 Poor positioning and/or body language

> **Clinician (standing at the foot of a patient's bed):** *"I'm sorry but we have had to cancel your discharge home."* Clinician then walks away.

In this scenario the clinician has not considered their own positioning or body language. They are standing away from the patient and above their eye level. There is no attempt to connect with the patient and explore the impact of the delayed discharge with them. The fact that the clinician then walks away and does not give the patient the opportunity to ask questions or clarify may result in a uninformed and confused patient.

How clinicians position themselves and what their body language is doing can have a negative impact on patients. This also links to eye contact. Often, we see clinicians looking at computer screens or notes when talking with patients.

 Time to think

> Think of a situation when someone is talking to you but not looking at you. It could be someone who is looking at a computer screen or a mobile phone. Consider how this made you feel. Based upon your thoughts, now consider if you ever talk to people but do not make eye contact or stand over them. How do you think this makes the person feel? Make your own notes here.
>
> _____
>
> _____
>
> _____
>
> _____

4.4 Avoidance of questions

Clinician: *"The scan shows your cancer has progressed... I will refer you to the Macmillan nurse"*. Clinician then walks away.

Kaye (2023) calls this the "hit and run", where clinicians deliver bad news then pass the buck to others to address the emotional fallout, rather than supporting the patient themselves and giving them time to absorb the information and ask questions. Unfortunately, this approach does not allow for clarification or explanation, and robs the patient of the opportunity to express emotion and to ask questions. One reason for this is that the healthcare professional may feel they do not have the time, knowledge or ability to deal with the emotion.

4.5 Not understanding or clarifying the patient's question

> **Relative:** *"Can you tell me where Mr Brown is please?"*
>
> **Clinician:** *"They've gone to Rose Cottage."* (colloquial name for mortuary)
>
> **Relative:** *"OK, when will he be back?"*

This is an example of when the clinician has answered the question correctly but has not considered the impact on the relative. Clearly the relative had not been informed at this point that Mr Brown had died. The healthcare practitioner should have taken the relative to a quiet room or location and established who they were, what they knew about the patient, then gently informed them that he had died.

4.6 Brushing over the concern

> **Patient:** *"Am I dying?"*
>
> **Clinician:** *"Well we are all dying. I could step out of here and be hit by a bus."*

For a patient to ask this question, they will have spent some time potentially plucking up the courage to ask. They may already have some insight into their illness; therefore, it is important to explore this with the patient. A more appropriate response would be to find out what has prompted the question. A possible response would be "*That must have been a difficult question for you to ask; what has prompted you to ask it now?*". In this scenario patients will often report signs and symptoms that could indicate that their suspicions are correct. Healthcare professionals can then use this information to confirm their suspicions (if true).

You can see from these scenarios that there was no thought and planning, nor empathy or consideration in delivering the news. Unfortunately, we still hear stories from patients recalling times when they were given bad news poorly and the negative impact of this. Ways to avoid these pitfalls are addressed in the next chapter where the mnemonic SUPPORTS is introduced, together with step-by-step guidance on how to use it.

 Notes

How to break bad news well – SUPPORTS model and steps

This new model/mnemonic has been developed by the author to help healthcare professionals structure their delivery of bad news, and consists of eight steps. The model is represented by a mnemonic as an aide-memoire: SUPPORTS.

SUPPORTS stands for

S: Set the scene

U: Understand the patient's perspective

P: Prepare the patient (fire a warning shot)

P: Pass on the information

O: Observe silence

R: Respect and respond to emotion

T: Time for questions and clarification

S: Summary and close

Each step will be addressed, offering information regarding the importance of the step.

5.1 S: Set the scene

When we know we will be delivering bad news, it is important to plan.

Factors that we need to take into consideration:

- Environment. Where are you going to deliver the bad news? Giving sensitive information in a busy ward environment is not good practice. Try to locate a quiet room or space away from other patients and busy environments.

- Consider your body language. Egan (1975) set out another mnemonic, SOLER, to aid clinicians' communication skills.
    - S: Sit squarely (45–80°; **not directly facing as this is confrontational**). Ensure you are at the same level as the patient and close to them (approx. 1½ × arm's length)
    - O: Open posture (don't cross your arms and legs)
    - L: Lean slightly forward (conveys empathy); Look genuinely interested; Listen attentively
    - E: Eye contact (but don't stare)
    - R: Remain relatively relaxed

Egan (2021)

- Ensure you have tissues *discreetly* available in the room within easy reach, should they be required.
- Time. Delivering bad news requires healthcare professionals to give the patient and/or relative the time to absorb the information and ask any questions they may have. Those receiving bad news often require time to understand the information, identify how the news may impact upon them, and formulate questions; therefore they should not feel rushed.
- Identify who is present. Does the patient want others to be around? Often it is helpful for patients to have a significant other present to hear the news too, to support them or to take notes.
- Avoid interruptions. Turn your phone/pager to silent. Put a 'Do not disturb' sign on the door.
- Know all the facts. It is important that we have all the information we are going to deliver ready. Update yourself with the notes and read any reports relating to the patient's condition.

5.2 U: Understand the patient's perspective

Establish early in the consultation what the patient's understanding is of the situation so far. You may recall telling them some news previously; however, we know that patients often don't hear/remember what they have been told previously (for a variety of reasons); therefore it is important to identify their perspective first.

If you know the patient well, this is an opportunity to check in with them regarding how they have been since your last review or conversation, e.g. *"How have you been since your last chemotherapy?"* or *"What do you recall from our last conversation?"* or *"Tell me what you understand regarding your health situation"*. This not only allows the practitioner to get information from the patient, but also allows the patient to feel heard and listened to, thus building up trust and rapport.

Listen to the words and phrases used. These words and phrases can be repeated back to demonstrate active listening, e.g. *"So you mention that you've not been sleeping well – tell me more about that. What has been keeping you awake?"*

5.3 P: Prepare (fire a warning shot)

Inform the patient that you have additional information to give, and seek permission to give it, e.g. *"I have the results of your latest scan – would you like me to go through that with you?"* Allow the patient thinking time to respond.

Denial or refusal to hear the news is a valid coping mechanism. For some patients the fear of bad news can be so overwhelming that they just aren't emotionally prepared to hear it. This should be explored further with the patient. Denial is discussed in *Section 5.11*.

Fire a second warning shot before you give the news, by stating that it is not good news or that it is bad news, e.g. *"I'm sorry but it is not good news"* then move on to give the information.

5.4 P: Pass on the information

Give the information in small pieces in a calm and slow manner. Do not rush to give all the news as quickly as you can – take your time.

Healthcare professionals are repeatedly criticised for using jargon and abbreviations. Ensure you use language that the patient will be able to understand. Some patients may be well informed and understand; however, we should never assume and should offer information in lay terms.

Some examples from clinical practice:

Jargon or medical term	Lay term
Orthopnoea	Breathlessness when lying down
Tachycardia	Fast heart rate
Peripheral oedema	Ankle swelling
Cellulitis	Skin infection
Hypotension	Low blood pressure

 Notes

_____

_____

_____

_____

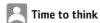 **Time to think**

Consider some of the terms and abbreviations you use in practice. How can you change your explanation, so that patients fully understand? Make your own notes here.

_____

_____

_____

_____

If there is more than one piece of information state this at the outset, e.g. *"I have three bits of information to go through with you"*, then deliver them one at a time. Some patients will not be able to cope with all the news in one sitting; if necessary, acknowledge that it is a lot to take in and schedule another appointment/time to continue.

Check understanding. This can be done at any point in the consultation and may be done during the 'time for questions' section.

5.5 O: Observe silence

Patients require time to process new information. Silence is one of the most powerful tools healthcare professionals can utilise. It allows patient thinking time. However, healthcare professionals say it is one of the most difficult things for them to master. It is natural to want to fill the silence; however, try to contain your desire to speak, and keep quiet.

Patients will eventually fill the silence, usually with a question or a statement to which we can respond. The art of good communication is also to be a good listener (Kaye, 2023). It is important that we not only listen to what the patient says when they break the silence, but also that we hear it and understand the meaning.

5.6 R: Respect and respond to emotion

Dealing with strong emotion is one of the biggest challenges healthcare professionals face and one that causes the greatest anxiety (Francis and Robertson, 2023).

Emotions when someone is given bad news can encompass anger, fear, frustration, crying, sadness, shock, guilt, etc. Kaye (2023) suggests that allowing patients to vent, followed by healthcare professionals "naming the emotion" facilitates the patient's ability to take some control.

Examples of a healthcare professional naming the emotion that they see would be "*I can see this news has made you upset*" or "*I can see you are shocked by this news*". By naming the emotion you are acknowledging that you can see the impact of the news you have delivered, and this display of empathy facilitates the building of a therapeutic relationship.

 Note of caution

> We should **never** say to a patient that we understand how they feel. Even if we have experienced something similar, this is unique to the individual and we can't possibly understand what this news means to them. Saying "*I understand*" can cause the opposite response to what we are trying to achieve. For some patients this can cause an increase in their anger.

5.7 T: Time for questions

Following the delivery of the news and dealing with the emotional impact, you should give patients the opportunity to ask any questions they may have. This allows for any misinterpretations to be corrected and allows for understanding to be reached.

There is no such thing as a 'silly question' and sometimes patients need permission to ask any questions about things they are unsure about. Also, despite telling a patient some information, they may not have taken it in due to anxiety, fear or simply just having too much information to remember it all. Giving patients the opportunity to ask questions and clarify ensures comprehension of the news and information.

We should also offer availability for when patients have had time to process the information but then have additional questions (see *Section 5.8*).

5.8 S: Summary and close

Healthcare professionals should close a consultation by summarising the key points and outlining a plan for what happens next. This may be awaiting further tests and investigations, referral to other services or scheduling a review.

Ensure you give patients contact information for either yourself (your service) or another point of contact should they have any additional questions or concerns. Kaye (2023) identifies that patients often need time for emotional adjustment and therefore may have questions or queries later that need addressing.

5.9 Example of using the mnemonic in practice

The following is a fictional transcript from a patient encounter that shows how the new SUPPORTS model can be used. It is worth adding that each encounter is different and unique, therefore listening to the patient's narrative and responding appropriately is key.

S: Set the scene

Prior to encounter: ensure a suitable location is used to deliver the information. Read the notes so you know the information you need to give to the patient or relative.

Ensure the furniture is positioned so the patient, relative and you are all at the same eye level.

Use the SOLER (Egan, 1975) acronym to set your body language correctly (see *Section 5.1*).

> **Clinician:** *"Hello Mrs Smith, come in and take a seat. My name is Lucy and I'm one of the specialist nurses. Who have you got with you today?"*
>
> **Patient:** *"Hello, please call me Mary. This is my son Peter."*
>
> **Clinician:** *"Welcome Peter. So, Mary, can you tell me how you have been since your last appointment?"*
>
> **Patient:** *"Oh I've been awful. I've been vomiting on and off for a few days now. My appetite has been really poor, and I feel like I've lost weight.*

U: Understand

Clinician: *"I'm sorry to hear that, Mary. I can help you with that but first I wanted to check with you what you understand about our appointment today. Do you know why you are here?"*

Patient: *"Yes, I'm here for my scan results."*

Clinician: *"Yes, that's my understanding too. So, what information do you recall from your last appointment?"*

Patient: *"I had been experiencing more pain so the doctor I saw last time thought it would be a good idea to have an up-to-date scan to see if my cancer has progressed. I'm really worried".*

Clinician: *"Tell me Mary, what is worrying you the most?"*

Patient: *"I'm worried that if the cancer has got worse that I won't be able to have any more chemotherapy".*

P: Prepare

Clinician: *"Well Mary, I do have your scan results. Would you like me to go through them with you?* (pause)

Patient: *"Well yes, I suppose so."*

Clinician: *"I'm sorry Mary, unfortunately it's not good news."* (pause)

P: Pass on the information

Clinician: *"Unfortunately the scan does show that your cancer has progressed."* (pause)

"We can see from the scan that the cancer is now in your liver."

O: Observe silence

At this point the clinician should remain quiet and allow the patient processing time. Maintain eye contact throughout.

R: Respect and respond to emotion

(Patient is gently crying)

Clinician: *"I can see this is upsetting for you and not the news you wanted to hear".*

Patient: *"I was worried that the cancer has progressed. I just knew 'cos I've been feeling so unwell."*

T: Time for questions

Clinician: *"Do you have any questions that you would like to ask?"*

Patient: *"Does that mean I can't have any more chemotherapy? Am I going to die soon?"*

Clinician: *"You've asked me two questions which I will try to address for you. In terms of the chemotherapy, I'll come back to that; however, you have asked a very difficult question... you ask if you are going to die soon. That's a difficult question to answer, but what has prompted you to ask it today?"*

Patient: *"My son is getting married next year. Do you think we should bring the wedding forward?"*

Clinician: *"Mary, it is really difficult to predict how long someone has left to live, but I can see this is really important to you to discuss. I think the thoughts you are having about bringing your son's wedding forward seem sensible given the circumstances."*

> Patient: *"Thank you for being honest. My son and I will discuss this over the next few days."*
>
> Clinician: *"Is there anything else you want to ask? Is there something else before we talk about treatment options?"*
>
> Patient: *"No, I just need to get my head around this."*

S: Summary and close

> Clinician: *"I can see this is a lot of information for you to take on board. We need to have a conversation regarding the treatment plan. Can I suggest we break here and come back together later to go through the options regarding ongoing treatment and symptom control."*
>
> Patient: *"Yes, thank you. That would be good."*

Although this is a brief encounter, you can see that the patient was given the information in an empathetic manner that allowed her to raise questions that were important to her. Some of the skills used by the clinician included 'parking', whereby they acknowledged a concern that needed addressing, but parked it with the intention of going back to it. Further information on skills and strategies can be found in *Chapter 6*.

As you familiarise yourself with the SUPPORTS model and start to use it in practice, you should also give further consideration to the following points.

5.10 Avoid assumptions

When delivering bad news, healthcare professionals should be inquisitive, using questioning to clarify points and to avoid making assumptions. Often, we assume patients know more than they do because we have assumed someone else has already told them, or we assume that because we told them 'last week' they can recall the information. Establishing the patient's perspective early in a consultation will give us insight into the patient's agenda. Neighbour (1987) advises that we need to establish the purpose of an encounter (or consultation) early and allow the patient to offer their narrative. Moulton (2016) discusses the 'golden minutes' whereby a health professional asks an open question such as *"How are you today?"* and allows the patient to speak uninterrupted. By utilising the 'golden minutes' it allows the patient to speak freely and gives the clinician some insight into the patient's problems. This approach facilitates the avoidance of assumptions and, with the use of further questions, can enable clinicians to understand the patient's perspective.

Scenario 1:

Clinician: *"I've brought you some lunch now that your surgery has been cancelled."*

Patient: *"What! No one has told me this... I'm nil by mouth."*

In this example the healthcare professional assumes that the patient has been informed that their surgery has been cancelled.

Scenario 2:

Clinician: *"Right, let's get this referral sorted for the Macmillan nurse to come and see you."*

Patient: *"What are you talking about? No one said I needed a Macmillan nurse."*

Clinician: *"Oh, Sally, the nurse you saw last week, said she told you she was going to make a referral."*

In this example the nurse had been told by her colleague that the patient already knew. One of two things could have happened here: either the patient didn't hear it (denial or anxiety) or Sally thought she had told them when in fact she hadn't.

Scenario 3:

Background: Patient A had undergone an emergency caesarean section and the baby was critically ill and taken to the neonatal intensive care unit (NICU), whilst the patient was taken to a maternity ward. The following day Patient A returns from visiting her newborn son on NICU to find a discharge letter placed on the bed.

> Patient: *"Nurse, why is this discharge letter on my bed?"*
>
> Clinician: *"Oh you can go home now."*
>
> Patient: *"But what about my baby? I don't want to leave him."*
>
> Clinician: *"Well, you can't stay in here indefinitely."*

In this scenario the patient was distressed at the prospect of having to leave her baby in hospital. No one took the time to explain or explore how she was feeling. For her the information was classed as bad news but was not considered to be so by the ward staff. There was an assumption that the patient was aware that she would be discharged without her baby.

5.11 Denial

Denial is a defence mechanism that some patients adopt unconsciously as a way of blocking out the reality of a difficult situation. Denial can be viewed negatively by healthcare professionals, but other theories exist that suggest denial allows for the pace of information delivery to be slowed down to a more manageable speed for the patient to be able to adapt to the situation (Kamen *et al.*, 2012). The fear from healthcare professionals when encountering patients in denial is that treatment options may be delayed and that communication channels between patients and clinicians can become blocked (Kogan *et al.*, 2013). Although the concept of denial is outside the scope of this book, it is important for clinicians to have an awareness of what it is and what purpose it serves. In terms of breaking bad news, it is suggested that when faced with a patient who is showing signs of being in denial, consider exploring this further. Healthcare professionals should explore the denial to determine if it is a total obstruction to understanding. If this is the case, then forcing a patient to hear the news could lead to severe psychological problems.

When you are following the SUPPORTS model, a patient may use denial and stop the flow of discussion at the 'P: Prepare the patient (fire a warning shot)' stage, as they are not ready to hear the news. This should be respected and explored further, as detailed below.

Notes

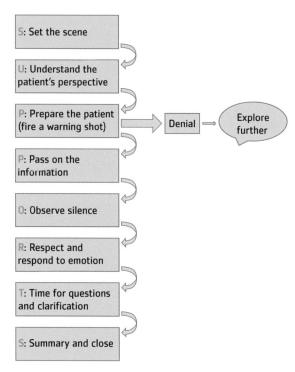

Key points in exploring denial include:

- Look for evidence that denial is not absolute (a window):
    Now – *"How do you feel things are going currently?"*
    Past – *"Has there ever been a time when you thought things weren't going to work out?"*
    Future – *"Have you got any concerns regarding your future in terms of your health?"*

If a patient displays complete denial of a situation, it is important to allow this to occur and to arrange for regular follow-up to reassess.

5.12 Therapeutic relationship and trust

When delivering bad news, clinicians should strive to build the therapeutic relationship to improve the experience for patients. Wright (2021) has a useful aide-memoire to assist clinicians:

ATTACH: how to develop a therapeutic relationship

- Authentic – be authentic with service users
- Trustworthy – be a reliable and well-informed professional so service users trust you, your judgement and your practice
- Time-maker – make time to be with service users, which makes them feel cared for and listened to, and enables professionals to discuss the time frame of care, including the ending of the therapeutic relationship
- Approachable – be approachable and visible, a good listener and provide empathetic responses
- Consistent – provide a consistent message, work as part of a team within recognised models of practice and within the requirements of the Nursing and Midwifery Council
- Honest – have open and realistic conversations with service users.

Patient satisfaction is improved when a therapeutic relationship is established.

6 Useful additional skills and strategies in communication

The following skills and strategies have been adapted from the Connected Advanced Communication Skills programme initially developed by Maguire *et al.* (1996) and advocated within the NHS Cancer Plan (DoH, 2000).

Silences

Eide *et al.* (2004) state that silences encourage people to say more about themselves and their predicament. When asked, many healthcare professionals report feeling uncomfortable using silence and say that they themselves want to fill the gaps in conversation. However, using silence is a powerful tool as it allows patients (or relatives/carers) to have thinking time and often, they will speak and offer insight into what they are thinking.

Phrases such as *"You appear to be thinking about something, can you tell me what is on your mind?"* may help as a stimulus to continue.

Encouragement

Encouragement can come in many forms. Things like using nods and ums and ahhs (called conversational fillers) act to encourage the person to keep talking. Equally phrases such as *"Go on"* or *"Tell me more"* will have the same effect.

Active listening

Active listening is said to be the art of hearing what a person has said whilst being able to withhold our own assumptions

(NHS England, 2021). Sometimes we can be guilty of not listening fully because we are formulating a response before the person has finished speaking. The skill of active listening requires healthcare professionals to not only hear the words but to understand their meaning. True active listening requires concentration.

Acknowledgement

One of the ways to demonstrate empathy is to acknowledge a person's emotion. Using phrases such as *"I can see you are saddened by the news"* or *"I can see this news has come as quite a shock"* allows the person you are communicating with to see that you can see the impact the news has had on them.

Reflection/paraphrasing

This tool encourages people to talk about an issue that they have raised indirectly; for example they may say *"I've been lying awake at night worrying"*. Healthcare practitioners can reflect the actual words used back to the patient, e.g. *"You say you have been lying awake worrying.... what is worrying you the most?"* or *"What have you been worrying about?"*. Sometimes patients will drop a hint that there is something concerning them, without actually saying it explicitly. Using the words and paraphrasing or reflecting the words displays that you have heard them and offers a window of opportunity to explore further.

Summarising

Patients quite often come with lots of problems. One way to ensure you have covered everything is to summarise the discussion and check for accuracy.

e.g. *"So, Mrs Smith, you tell me you are worried about your treatment options, pain in your back and that you are worried about how you will manage looking after your husband. Which one of these concerns would you like to address first?"*

In this example the clinician has summarised back what the patient has said. You can then ask which problem they would like to address first. This may also be combined with 'parking', as discussed later.

Empathy

Empathy and sympathy are different concepts. You can display empathy by using phrases such as *"It sounds like things have been really difficult for you"* without saying you understand.

 Note

> Clinicians should avoid using the phrase *"I understand"*. You can never truly understand what the patient is going through; even if you have experienced it yourself or cared for many patients with a similar concern, it will be different for that person and can never truly be the same.

Educated guess

An educated guess is sometimes required if you have a gut instinct that something is occurring and yet the patient hasn't explicitly told you.

An example might be *"From what you are saying I'm guessing you have a lot on your plate... is that correct?"*

It can be a useful strategy to use when you want to explore something, and allows the patient or relative to confirm or refute the suggestion. It also allows you to display empathy, in that you have picked up on something that has been implied rather than explicitly said.

Challenging

Sometimes patients say words that don't seem to match what their body language is saying. For example, a patient might be displaying signs that they are agitated yet saying they are 'fine'. Using a phrase such as *"I know you say you are fine, but I can't help but sense that perhaps you aren't. Can we talk about what is making you so unsettled?"*.

'Parking'

Quite often patients will raise more than one concern at a time. This can be challenging to manage; however, one strategy is to use 'parking'. Acknowledge the concern and 'park it' so you can address something else, then come back to it. At the summary and close, ask the patient if you have covered everything that was raised, ensuring that the concepts that were 'parked' have been covered. Alternatively, if you do not have time to address every concern raised on this occasion, acknowledge them all, repeating them back, e.g. *"So you've said you are worried about X, Y and Z. As we are limited for time, which would you like me to focus our time on today? We can revisit the others another time."*

Chunk and check

Chunk and check is a skill that encourages healthcare practitioners, who are required to give a lot of information, to break it into small bite-sized pieces. As previously mentioned, patients often only recall the first and last thing they were told. By breaking down the news or information into smaller pieces and checking understanding before moving on, the patient's recall of all the information is facilitated.

Additional helpful phrases

These are some phrases and questions that I have found helpful. You can add to this notes page phrases that you find useful yourself in practice.

"I've been asked to come and talk to you by your doctor, and they have given me some information about you, but before we start, I'd like you to explain to me in your own words what's been happening."

"That's a really difficult question. Can I ask what has made you ask that today?"

"Can I check, what have you been told already?"

"Did anyone explain what that meant?"

"Do you have any thoughts or concerns about your future that you would like to discuss?"

"I would like to talk to you about a difficult topic... would that be OK?"

"What is worrying you the most?"

_____

_____

_____

_____

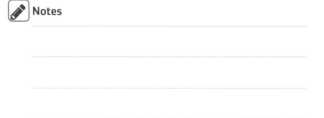

Notes

Within this book, there is acknowledgement of the challenges faced by healthcare professionals who are called upon to deliver bad news. Each patient encounter is unique and the way in which the patient responds is unique. However, the use of the new model/mnemonic adds structure and acts as a guide to assist practitioners when delivering bad news.

The underlying principles in breaking bad news are to take a patient-centred approach and to involve patients in the discussion, allowing them time to absorb the information and to ask questions.

Final word – look after yourself

Working in health care is rewarding as well as being challenging at times, and we have all finished a shift and 'taken the patient home' mentally. Neighbour (1987) advocates 'housekeeping' within his consultation model; or in other words, looking after yourself and being ready for the next patient. Being the deliverer of bad news can be a major source of stress, anxiety and burnout for clinicians, with Moulton (2016) suggesting that each consultation requires us to give a little bit of ourselves; this is particularly true when delivering bad news. We are humans, with feelings, emotions and our own vulnerabilities which need nurturing and looking after. Freeman (2015) acknowledges that looking after oneself can be difficult and something we often neglect; however, she advocates for clinicians to consider self-care daily, suggesting clinicians identify sources of support, both within the workplace – for example peer supervision, group supervision, debriefing sessions, etc. – and away from work, such as practising mindfulness or other de-stressing activities.

References

Almaguer, A., Garcia, I., Arnaud, D. *et al.* (2017) Are we prepared to give bad news? An international survey analysis. *Chest*, **152(4):** A836.

Buckman, R. (1984) Breaking bad news: why is it still so difficult? *British Medical Journal (Clin Res Ed)*, **288:** 1597–9.

Calnan, M. and Rowe, R. (2008) *Trust Matters in Health Care.* Open University Press.

Cheon, S., Fu, W., Agarwal, A., Henry, B. and Chow, E. (2017) The impact of breaking bad news on oncologist burnout and how communication skills can help: a scoping review. *Journal of Pain Management*, **10(1):** 89–97.

Connolly, M., Perryman, J., McKenna, Y. *et al.* (2010) SAGE & THYME: a model for training health and social care professionals in patient-focussed support. *Patient Education and Counseling*, **79:** 87–93.

Department of Health (2000) *The NHS Cancer Plan.* DoH.

Edwards, M. (2010) How to break bad news and avoid common difficulties. *Nursing and Residential Care*, **12(10):** 495–7.

Egan, G. and Reese, R.J. (2021) *The Skilled Helper: a client-centred approach*, 3rd EMEA edition. Cengage.

Eide, H., Quera, V., Graugaard, P. and Finset, A. (2004) Physician–patient dialogue surrounding patients' expression of concern: applying sequence analysis to RIAS. *Social Science & Medicine*, **59(1):** 145–55.

Epstein, R., Borrell, F. and Caterina, M. (2000) *Communication and Mental Health in Primary Care.* Oxford University Press.

Fallowfield, L., Jenkins, V., Farewell, V. *et al.* (2002) Efficacy of a Cancer Research UK communication skills training model for oncologists: a randomised controlled trial. *The Lancet*, **359(9307):** 650–6.

Fallowfield, L. and Jenkins, V. (2004) Communicating sad, bad, and difficult news in medicine. *The Lancet*, **363(9405):** 312–19.

Fox B.M. (2021) Looking behind the fear of becoming a burden. *HEC Forum*, **33:** 401–14.

Francis, L. and Robertson, N. (2023) Healthcare practitioners' experiences of breaking bad news: a critical interpretative meta synthesis. *Patient Education and Counseling*, **107:** 107574.

Freeman, B. (2015) *Compassionate Person-centred Care for the Dying: an evidence-based palliative care guide for nurses.* Springer.

Glanzer, M. and Cunitz, A.R. (1966) Two storage mechanisms in free recall. *Journal of Verbal Learning and Verbal Behavior*, **5(4):** 351–60.

Greenhalgh, T. and Heath, I. (2010) *Measuring Quality in the Therapeutic Relationship.* King's Fund.

Heaven, C.M. and Maguire, P. (1997) Disclosure of concerns by hospice patients and their identification by nurses. *Palliative Medicine*, **11(4):** 283–90.

Kamen, C., Taniguchi, S., Student, A. *et al.* (2012) The impact of denial on health-related quality of life in patients with HIV. *Quality of Life Research*, **21(8):** 1327–36.

Kaye, P. (1996) *Breaking Bad News: a ten-step approach* (1st edition). EPL Publications.

Kaye, P. (2023) *Breaking Bad News: a ten-step approach* (updated edition). Scion Publishing Ltd.

Kogan, N.R., Dumas, M. and Cohen, S.R. (2013) The extra burdens patients in denial impose on their family caregivers. *Palliative & Supportive Care*, **11(2)**: 91–9.

Maguire, P., Booth, K., Elliott, C. and Jones, B. (1996) Helping health professionals involved in cancer care acquire key interviewing skills – the impact of workshops. *European Journal of Cancer*, **32A(9)**: 1486–9.

Mirhaghi, A., Sharafi, S., Bazzi, A. and Hasanzadeh, F. (2017) Therapeutic relationship: is it still heart of nursing? *Nursing Reports* (Pavia, Italy), **7(1)**.

Monden, K.R., Gentry, L. and Cox, T.R. (2016) Delivering bad news to patients. *Baylor University Medical Center Proceedings*, **29(1)**: 101–2.

Moreno-Poyato, A.R. and Rodríguez-Nogueira, Ó. (2021) The association between empathy and the nurse–patient therapeutic relationship in mental health units: a cross-sectional study. *Journal of Psychiatric and Mental Health Nursing*, **28(3)**: 335–43.

Moulton, L. (2016) *The Naked Consultation: a practical guide to primary care consultation skills* (2nd edition). CRC Press.

Murdock, B.B. (1962) The serial position effect of free recall. *Journal of Experimental Psychology*, **64(5)**: 482–8.

National Institute for Health and Care Excellence (2021) *Shared Decision Making*. NICE.

Neelima, Y., Begum, K.J., Ali, S.A. *et al.* (2020) Perceived barriers of communication between nurses and patients in a tertiary care hospital. *Indian Journal of Public Health Research & Development*, **11(7)**: 1009–15.

Neighbour, R. (1987) *The Inner Consultation*. MTP Press Ltd.

NHS Digital (2022) *Data on Written Complaints in the NHS 2020–21*. Available at: https://digital.nhs.uk/data-and-information/publications/statistical/data-on-written-complaints-in-the-nhs

NHS England (2012) *Compassion in Practice*. NHS England.

NHS England (2021) *Active Listening*. NHS England and NHS Improvement.

Norouzinia, R., Aghabarari, M., Shiri, M., Karimi, M. and Samami, E. (2015) Communication barriers perceived by nurses and patients. *Global Journal of Health Science*, **8(6)**: 65–74.

Spiers, J.A. and Wood, A. (2010) Building a therapeutic alliance in brief therapy: the experience of community mental health nurses. *Archives of Psychiatric Nursing*, **24(6)**: 373–386.

Wilkinson, S., Linsell, L., Perry, R. and Blanchard, K. (2008) Effectiveness of a three-day communication skills course in changing nurses' communication skills with cancer/palliative care patients: a randomised controlled trial. *Palliative Medicine*, **22(4)**: 365–75.

Wright, K.M. (2021) Exploring the therapeutic relationship in nursing theory and practice. *Mental Health Practice*, **24(5)**: 34–41.

Further reading

Collini, A., Parker, H. and Oliver, A. (2021) Training for difficult conversations and breaking bad news over the phone in the emergency department. *Emergency Medicine Journal*, **38:** 151–4.

Edwards, S., Keillor, L., Sandison, L., Millett, A. and Davies, F. (2021) 50 Time critical telephone conversations in the emergency department – a pilot educational project to improve communication skills over the telephone when breaking bad news to relatives. *BMJ Supportive & Palliative Care*, **11:** A26–A27.

Kornhaber, R., Walsh, K., Duff, J. and Walker, K. (2016) Enhancing adult therapeutic interpersonal relationships in the acute healthcare setting: an integrative review. *Journal of Multidisciplinary Healthcare*, **9:** 537–46.

My Notes

My Notes